GW00746399

Your New Grandchild

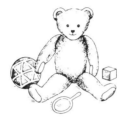

A collection by
BARTY PHILLIPS

PIATKUS

The poems by Emma Bosely (page 13), Gail Bloomfield (page 25), Paul Leipnik (page 34) and Andrew Darley (page 58) appear by permission of W H Smith & Sons; they have all been award-winning entries in their Young Writers' Competitions. The poem by John Kitching (page 21) appears by permission of the author.

With many thanks to Kathleen Le Mare for her experience and advice, and to Keith Shepherd for his birthday card.

First published in Great Britain in 1988 by
Judy Piatkus (Publishers) Limited of
5 Windmill Street, London W1P 1HF

British Library Cataloguing in Publication Data

Phillips, Barty
Your new grandchild : a collection.
1. Babies
I. Title
305.2'32

ISBN 0-86188-767-0

Designed by Sue Ryall
Cover artwork by Sue Warne

Phototypeset in Linotron Melior by
Phoenix Photosetting, Chatham
Printed and bound in Great Britain at
The Bath Press, Avon

CONTENTS

iii

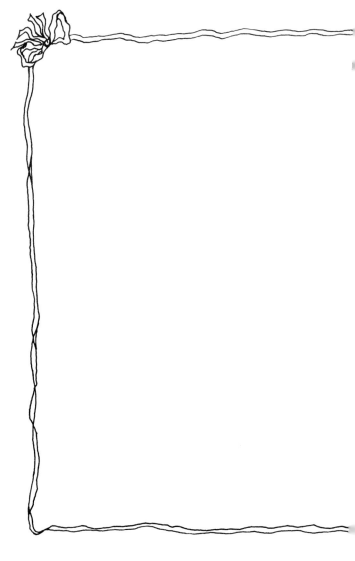

GRANDMOTHER'S GARDEN

I went into my Grandmother's garden,
And there I found a farthing.
I went into my next-door neighbour's;
There I bought a pipkin, a popkin,
A slipkin and a slopkin
A nailboard, a sailboard,
And all for a farthing.

Traditional nursery rhyme

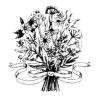

MY GRANDDAUGHTER

My granddaughter is beautiful. When she was born
she was blonde and long and leggy and the image of
her father's side of the family. Now she's six with
long dark hair, she looks just like her mother, my
daughter. And she is still like her father's side of the
family too.

She has the biggest blue eyes I have ever seen and a
determined personality. That is to say, she knows
what she likes and in her quiet way will get it. She
likes pretty things and peaceful things. She likes to
think about what she wants to say before she says it.
She likes things to be neat and tidy and she likes
pretty clothes – she won't wear tracksuits or jeans
and her shoes must be shiny. She has a cake tin full
of beads and bits of costume jewellery and she will
be happy for hours squatting by the front door
playing with them and swirling around in her
mother's scarves.

My granddaughter has always had sophisticated
tastes in food. She likes olives and prawns and
avocados. She likes to think she is a fairy princess.

My granddaughter makes me proud to be a
grandmother. She has removed from me the fear of
growing old. She is my companion and my friend. I
hope she knows this. I think she is sure to.

GRANDPARENTING IN THE EIGHTIES

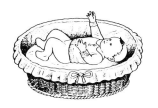

Grandparents in the eighties are not the little old people with sticks and beaked noses and gnarled fingers they were of yore. They are people on the brink of a new life that has lots to offer them. Their grandchildren present new opportunities for friendship, and exploration of the modern world – which grandchildren may well help their grandparents to understand. The modern grandparent may be Dallas-shouldered and ready for a sophisticated day at the office, or red-tracksuited to go roller-skating with the grandchildren.

Grandchildren can derive a sense of place, of knowing who they are, from listening to their grandparents talk about their past and their experiences, their family and childhood. Particularly when they are small, children can get a sense of continuity and family by looking at photographs and mementos of their own mother or father when young.

The embargo on physical closeness which sometimes exists in the relationship with a son or daughter is often lifted in the relationship with the grandchildren. Grandfathers seem to enjoy flirting with their growing-up granddaughters and grandmothers will often become quite young and flighty when their grandsons make a fuss of them. Grandparents should delight in this very special relationship.

There is also, in a technological and fast-moving age, a good chance that you will be able to let your grandchildren teach you a thing or two – about computers, say, or some other electronic device which they feel at home with. Why not get your grandchild to educate you into the mysteries of using a word processor, setting up a video recorder or playing computer games? Just a little ignorance can always be assumed, though the chances are that you really will not know how the thing works!

If you find your new role as a grandparent difficult at first, you are certainly not alone. One young mother says: 'For some reason my mother became absolutely cold-ridden as soon as she had to confront my child. She couldn't cross the room; she would sneeze; she would blow her nose; she couldn't pick up the kid – and the same thing happened with her second grandchild, my younger sister's. She couldn't come near the child. She said to me, when I asked her about it later on, "How did I know what I would feel as a grandmother? I didn't know if I would like my grandchild."' (From an interview by Judith Arcana in *Our Mothers' Daughters*, published by The Women's Press.)

What's more, it's easy to stereotype oneself. When my first grandchild was born I went out and bought myself a suit. Not until I got it home did I realise that I'd bought one which in the back of my mind I had labelled 'suitable for grandmothers'. It was dull brown, tweedy and sensible. I have never worn it.

Old people often say that they notice changes in their own attitudes towards young children as the years go by. 'As a person gets older I definitely think he gets more love for children,' one London grandfather said.

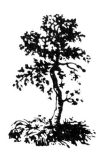

BABOUSCHKA

The Russians have a story about Babouschka
(Granny). Everyone was watching for a star – except
Babouschka. She was too busy sweeping, cooking
and gardening. So when it came, she missed the
twinkling star; nor did she hear the pipes and the
drums and the tinkling of bells. But she couldn't miss
the knocking.

'Now what?' she said, opening the door. There
were three Kings and a servant.

'Come with us,' said the Kings.

'But I haven't anything for him.'

'Give him some of your pickle, it's very good,' said
the Kings.

'Nonsense, that's not for a baby,' said Babouschka.

The Kings waved goodbye. When they had gone
she thought sadly of her cupboard full of toys for her
boy, who died when he was very small. After she had
tidied and swept and washed up, beaten the cushions
and washed the clothes, at last she went to the small
cupboard and brought out the toys, all dusty,
certainly not fit for a King. She worked and worked,
cleaning the wooden reindeer, the wooden polar
bears, the wooden pipes, and the little Russian
Babouschka doll in her own image. Then she was so
tired that she fell asleep.

Suddenly she woke up and rushed out. No star.
She put on her cloak and hurried through village

after village. Everybody she met had seen the Kings –
they went that way. The villages became towns. Then
a city.

After days and days she got to Bethlehem. 'Yes,'
said the people, 'the Kings were here and the
shepherds too; and yes, they saw the Christ Child,
the saviour of the world. Here's the stable where he
was. Now they've gone to Egypt. You are too late.'

Babouschka is still looking for the Christ Child.
She goes from house to house saying, 'Is he here? Is
he here?' At Christmas, when she sees a sleeping
child, she lifts out a toy from her basket and leaves it,
just in case.

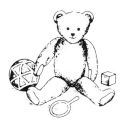

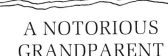

A NOTORIOUS GRANDPARENT

Of all the notorious grandparents in history, Elizabeth, Empress of Russia from 1741 to 1762, probably takes the cake. She was the daughter of Peter the Great and mother-in-law of Catherine the Great. When Catherine's first son Paul was born, Elizabeth made sure that the birth took place in her own apartments. Catherine wrote: 'No sooner had the baby been born, baptised and swaddled than the Empress ordered the midwife to take the child and follow her.'

The Empress took the baby to her own room, 'and the moment he cried, she rushed and literally smothered him with her attentions'. The room was kept excessively hot and the baby was swaddled in flannel, laid in a cot lined with silver fox, and covered with a padded satin quilt over which was placed another counterpane of pink velvet lined with silver fox. He was often bathed in sweat from head to foot.

Catherine was not allowed to see her baby again for well over a month. Then, she wrote: 'The Empress came a second time to my room for the churching ceremony. This was the first time I had seen him since his birth. I found him beautiful and the sight of him made my heart rejoice, but the moment the prayers were over, the Empress had him carried away, and herself departed.'

A GRANDSON'S BIRTHDAY GREETING

When ten-year-old Keith was not well his grandmother used to go and play cards with him to keep him entertained. They got on really well together, sometimes playing for fun and sometimes for small bets, building up a cowboy saloon atmosphere together. When his grandmother's birthday arrived he took great pains to make her a birthday card which said:

'Here's a birthday greeting to the . . . FASTEST NANA IN THE WEST!'

Inside there was a poem which read:

'There once was a Nana
The best in the town,
She shot a six shooter
Like an old Texas Ranger,
20 young cowboys had tried her and failed.

Cards were her magic
And no one could beat her
All the best played her
Until they could keep up the stakes no more.

The Best she was
And The Best she'll stay.'

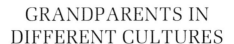

GRANDPARENTS IN
DIFFERENT CULTURES

The world over, a grandmother will have useful lore
to offer about cooking and housewifery, if only
because she has been at it so much longer than others
in the family.

Chinese culture demands a great deal of
self-discipline from the age group who are parents
but is lenient towards the social foibles of children
and old people. Parents may not express their
feelings in public, but grandparents and
grandchildren are able to get up to all sorts of things
and no one remonstrates with them about their odd
behaviour. Chinese grandparents are greatly
respected by their children and grandchildren, and it
is very common for three generations to live together.
If they don't, then the grandmothers and grandfathers
will take turns to visit their children and stay with
them for about a week at a time.

Older members of Japanese families often have a
display altar which can be opened up. Grandchildren
bring offerings such as fruit or cakes to remember
members of the family who have died. Grandmothers
may make paper dolls in traditional Japanese style
and give classes in paper crafts to local people.

In Italy families are also close. Grandchildren pay
frequent visits to their grandparents. The great
festival is Easter when the family will go to the

grandparents for Easter dinner and enjoy a special cake shaped like a cross.

In Egypt the grandmother will make goat's cheese for the whole family and also perhaps sell it in the village dairy. She may keep ducks in a small pen and have dovecotes built of mud. She makes a week's supply of bread at a time and buys most of the family food from street traders who come right to her door loaded with goods on donkeys or on wooden barrows. She will share the cooking with the younger women. The grandmother is an important influence; in fact the wishes of both grandparents must be obeyed even in the most modern Egyptian homes.

Families in the modern industrial-based countries of the West are more likely to be split up, so that grandparents have less day-to-day influence. But they can provides treats and interesting holidays, and an understanding and sympathetic 'ear' by either letter, tape or telephone.

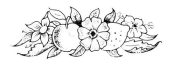

Some names for grandparents

Granny and Grandad	English
Dama-wyn and Hendas	Cornish
Nain and Taid	Welsh
Nonna and Nonno	Italian
Oma and Opa	German/Dutch
Bedstemoder and Bedstefader	Danish
Bonne-maman and Grandpapa	French
Avia and Avus	Latin
Abuelita and Abuelito	Spanish
Babouschka and Deduschka	Russian
Por-por and Kung-kung	Cantonese
Nenek and Nenek	Malay

'You no done breed, so you no laugh after your grannie.'

Jamaican proverb

WHEN MY NANA
ABANDONED ME

I had made camps under their table
And dished up pretend food on plastic plates.
Papa would take me to Stumpy Park:
There was a huge log that I used to stand on.

I would come back and play in the sandpit:
It was at the bottom of the garden.
Papa had made it just for me.
It was good for studying ant life.

In the summer I'd sit outside in my mini garden chair
Sipping lemonade and eating fly biscuits.
There were numerous apple trees in their garden
And I would enjoy wheeling my baby wheelbarrow
Collecting apples that had dropped to the ground.

When Nana and Papa took me to Carner Park
We'd have a picnic and then play ball.
All sorts of dogs stole my ball.
Papa had to run off to rescue it.
When I was tired
Nana let me ride on her lap in the wheelchair.

On cold days I played with Nana's silk scarves
Or my Papa helped me make Dougals
Out of wool and pingpong balls.

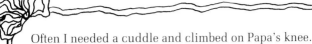

Often I needed a cuddle and climbed on Papa's knee.
I had to be careful:
He'd had a car accident
And hurt his chest.

In the afternoon my Papa would doze.
Nana and I disappeared into the kitchen
And got out the paint pots.
We had to take it in turns:
There was only one brush.
Nana had a candle:
I made magic pictures with it.

When they both nodded off
I trundled into the bedroom
To investigate Nana's jewellery.

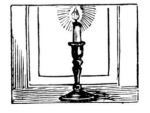

Now and again clothes catalogues
Came through the door.
I snuggled up to Nana,
We both liked clothes.

My favourite books were about Old Lob.
Nana read them to me.
And she taught me how to draw pigs
With big, fat, chunky crayons.

Then suddenly when I was eight
My Nan died.
I felt empty and sad.
Would my Mum die too?
My Papa felt lost as well for a long time.
I still cry inside.

Emma Bosely (aged 13), from
Young Words 1986 (Macmillan)

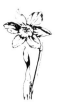

GRANDPARENTS IN CHILDREN'S LITERATURE

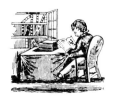

Victorian children's literature was full of grumpy old grandparents who disowned their daughters for marrying unsuitable men and were then won over by the sweet ways and wiles of their grandchildren. In this vein Juliana Horatia Ewing wrote a story called *The Peace Egg* in which children didn't realise that the cross old man next door was their grandfather, until his heart was softened when they acted a play for him.

Frances Hodgson Burnett created, in the same genre, Little Lord Fauntleroy – a too-good-to-be-true lad who was summoned from poverty in America to be brought up by his noble grandfather. Grandfather would not speak to his daughter and housed her in a lodge at the bottom of the drive. (Her offence had been to marry an American who had since died, of course.) Little Lord Fauntleroy's winning ways – and the threat of a pretender whom his grandfather detested – won the old man round.

Another grandparent grumpy to adults but understanding to children was the splendid Uncle Alp in Heidi, who managed to make his little granddaughter feel at home, even though she was landed on him out of the blue:

'Heidi picked up the bundle and followed the old man into a biggish room which was the whole extent of his living quarters. She saw a table and a chair, and his bed over in one corner. Opposite that was a stove, over which a big pot was hanging. There was a door in one wall which the old man opened, and she saw it was a large cupboard with his clothes hanging in it. There were shelves in it too. One held his shirts, socks and handkerchiefs, another plates, cups and glasses, while on the top one were a round loaf, some smoked meat, and some cheese. Here, in fact, were all the old man's possessions. Heidi went inside the open cupboard and pushed her bundle right away to the back so that it would not easily be seen again.

"Where shall I sleep, Grandfather?" she asked next.

"Where you like," he replied.

This answer pleased Heidi, and as she was looking round the room for a good place she noticed a ladder propped against the wall near her grandfather's bed. She climbed up it at once and found herself in a hay loft. A pile of fresh, sweet-smelling hay lay there, and there was a round hole in the wall of the loft, through which she could see right down the valley.

"I shall sleep here," she called down. "It's a

splendid place. Just come and see, Grandfather."

"I know it well," he called back.

"I'm going to make my bed now," she went on, "but you'll have to come up and bring me a sheet to lie on."

"All right," said the old man, "but it needs to be thicker than that," and he spread a lot more hay over hers so that she would not feel the hard floor.

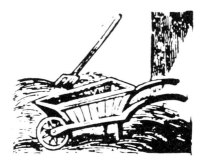

The thick cloth which he had brought for a sheet was so heavy that she could hardly lift it by herself, but its thickness made it a good protection against the prickly hay stalks. Together they spread it out, and Heidi tucked the ends under her "mattress" to make it all neat and comfortable. Then she looked at her bed thoughtfully for a moment and said, "We've forgotten something, Grandfather."

"What's that?"

"A blanket to cover it, so that I can creep under it when I go to bed."

"That's what you think, is it? Suppose I haven't got one?"

"Oh well then, it doesn't matter," said Heidi, "I can easily cover myself with hay," and she was just going to fetch some more when her grandfather stopped her.

"Wait a bit," said, and he went down the ladder, and took from his own bed a great sack made of heavy linen which he brought up to the loft. "There, isn't that better than hay?" he asked, as they put it over the bed.

Heidi was delighted with the result.

"That's a wonderful blanket, and my whole bed's lovely. I wish it was bedtime now so that I could get in it. . . ."

The wind was so strong, it almost blew her away, so she finished her bread and milk quickly and went indoors and up to bed. There she was soon sleeping as soundly as if she was tucked up in the finest bed in the world. Her grandfather went to bed also before it was dark, for he always got up with the sun, and that came over the mountain tops very early in the summer. During the night the wind blew so hard that it shook the whole hut and made its beams creak. It shrieked down the chimney and brought one or two of the old fir trees' branches crashing down. So after a while the old man got up, thinking, "The child may be frightened."

19

He climbed up the ladder and went over to her bed. Just then the moon, which had been covered by scudding clouds, shone straight through the hole in the wall on to Heidi's face. She was fast asleep under her heavy coverlet, one rosy cheek resting on her chubby little arm, and with such a happy expression on her face that she must surely have been dreaming of pleasant things. He stood looking down at her till clouds covered the moon again, darkening the room. Then he went back to bed.'

*

Modern fictional grandparents have a different way of impressing their grandchildren. In *The Granny Season* by Joan Phipson (Hamish Hamilton), Granny wins the day at the school cricket match, having played for the Australian women's team in her salad days. The traditional image of granny as timid, wispy and frail then vanishes from the small boy's mind as he is grudgingly but completely won over by this new-look grandparent.

'Only know that posterity is there when a grandson plays at the gate.'

Hindi proverb

GRAN

'My Goodness! What a big boy you are!
Good gracious! How you've grown!'
The first words always from my gran:
They always make me moan.

'You must have been drinking your milk up;
You must have been eating your greens;
You must have been going to bed early.'
I'm really fed up with these scenes.

Do you think I should tell her
How small she is? 'I do believe you've shrunk.
Why are you growing a beard Gran?
You're beginning to look like a monk.

'You must have been drinking the gin, Gran.
You eat too much pudding and cake,
You've been watching the Hulk on TV, Gran.
How about a quick jump in the lake?'

But no. I'll just grin it and bear it
And take growing pains like a man.
I'll kiss her moustache; hold my hand out –
And get pocket money from Gran.

John Kitching, from
A Second Poetry Book
(Oxford University Press)

GRANDPARENTS REMEMBERED

Many people have remembered their grandparents with special affection, and in the Russian writer Maxim Gorki's childhood his grandmother seems to have been the saving grace in a poverty-stricken and brutal upbringing.

'When she had somehow managed to disentangle her hair, she would quickly plait it into thick strands, hurriedly wash herself, snorting angrily, and then stand before her icons, without having succeeded in washing away the irritation from her large face, all wrinkled with sleep. And now would begin the real morning ablution which straight away completely refreshed her. She would straighten her stooping back, throw her head back and gaze lovingly at the round face of the Virgin of Kazan, throw her arms out wide, cross herself fervently and whisper noisily in heated voice:

   "Blessed Virgin, remember us in times of trouble . . ."

   Her dark eyes smiled and she seemed to grow younger again as she crossed herself again with slow movements of her heavy hand.'

From *My Childhood* (Penguin Classics)

Rabbi Lionel Blue, Convenor of the Reform Synagogue of Great Britain (and the Radio Four Rabbi) grew up in his grandmother's house in the East End of London in the thirties. Cabbage borscht was inevitably offered to all who came to the tiny terraced house in a street that has now gone. She ran open house, Russian-style, with a samovar and a table filled with food. The place was alive with endless people – White Russians, Polish, Yiddish, cockney – and the spirit of Eastern Europe. Until Lionel Blue was evacuated to Devon it never occurred to him that meals started and ended and that you invited people for dinner.

'She cooked because God wanted her to. He had said so in the scriptures and so she cooked! All her prayers had been answered: she had arrived safely in London . . . She was happy. So she cooked! . . . Her famous cabbage borscht illustrated to her the problem and the solution. Quantities were never exact; life was never exact.'

From *Taste* magazine, December/January 1988

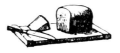

Bella Lyon was a strong-minded grandmother whose granddaughter, Helen Lyon Adamson, remembered her in her book *Grandmother's Household Hints* (Frederick Muller).

'Meet Bella Lyon. She stood five feet four in her size five shoes and was straight as a ramrod; she had small, square hands, an eighteen-inch waist and never wore a corset in her life; her chestnut hair was piled high upon her head in a rather elaborate coiffure; her eyes, large and pansy-brown, could show gleams of kindness as well as flinty glints of stubborn determination; her voice, low-pitched and clear, could ring with authoritative timbre . . . There was nothing her servants might be called upon to do she could not do herself, and perhaps, even a little better. In fact, when I was in my teens, I learned to thank my lucky stars that I was Bella's granddaughter, not her daughter, and therefore not exposed to her benevolent but militant domestic tyranny.'

'There will be no loving completely until the grandchild arrives.'

Eastern proverb

OLD GRANDMA

Her skin clung to the oldness
Of her hand like rose petals
Clothed in water.
She folded my hand in hers
And patted it softly.

She looked at me with the lustre of a diamond
In each eye.
Her hair was twined back into
A grey bun, swerving and
Curving its way round
Like soft smoke.

Her eyes wandered with thoughts
And stared at me.

I bent forward and kissed her wrinkled cheek.
It was like kissing clay,
All cold and soft.

I took a deep breath and smelled
Mint humbugs and golden fudges.
I began to feel saddened by the way she moved
Like a clock winding down,
Getting slower.

POOR OLD GRANDMA

Gail Bloomfield (aged 13),
from *Young Words 1986* (Macmillan)

MY GRANDSONS

I have two grandsons. They are both the same age: just three years old. They are very different in character, but seem to complement each other and always enjoy each other's company. The older one (by a month) is a tall boy with straight blond hair and a serious frown which can change to an enchanting and welcoming smile. He is solid and methodical. He stomps along in a determined way and will patiently study anything he's interested in until he understands its workings. He does not suffer fools gladly – child or adult. One of his greatest treats is being given a ride in a friend's sports car. His face lights up with pleasure and this friend is his idol.

The other boy is a piece of quicksilver. He is small and neat for his age and very speedy and sure on his feet. He has twinkling almond-shaped eyes – goodness knows where they come from. I don't know anybody else in the family with eyes like that, except his father at the same age. He has an appetite like a little bird and it is the family hobby to try to get him to eat. He is impatient and wants to be able *to do* things immediately. When frustrated, he flings his toys right across the room and shrieks loud and piercingly. He loves the big muddy puddle in the lane outside my house and his parents have to bring extra clothes when they visit because we all know he is going to march straight into it when he gets here.

I took the boys to a Punch and Judy show when they were two years old. At the end of the performance both children had disappeared. The older one was discovered round the back of the booth trying to unravel the puppet master's secrets and mysteries; the other had disappeared right out of the hall with the departing audience.

Both boys, the one thoughtful and determined, the other emotional and passionate, delight in each other's company. They may lock in silent battle over the right to ride the tricycle and screech over ownership of a favourite model car, but secretly each admires and is amused by the other. They are always happy on the days when they are going to see each other again.

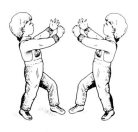

ST. JOHN'S CHURCH

The tower tall stands by the wall
And stands there day and night.
It is a lovely sight.
The wall is long
Bells sing their song
And carols rise in the skies
People sing and church bells ring
They sing and church bells ring.

(I wrote this poem for my granny.)

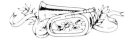

BOOKS TO READ WITH YOUR GRANDCHILDREN

Being read to can be a rare treat for the very young; but if you can tell your own stories, this is magic. Many parents have reason to be grateful to their own parents for entertaining the grandchildren with stories about particular people – my own father's to my children were about Mr. Postlethwaite, his granddaughter Feather and their dog Pie; or stories which have the same familiar ending – such as a policeman's whiskers catching fire; or stories that actually happened – about grandfather's extraordinary schooldays or grandmother's equally extraordinary courtship.

'When I got my first bustle, I had to keep peering round to see if it was wagging properly,' one grandmother remembers *her* grandmother recalling. The sailor who eventually married the young lady with the bustle had equally fascinating tales to tell his grandchildren – about being on the tea clippers, of bubonic plague on the high seas, and being lashed to the wheel in a storm.

Books, too, can be magic. It is useful for grandparents to keep a bookshelf or suitcase of books that grandchildren can help themselves to while in the house but may not take home. Much of the charm of 'Granny's Special Books' is the fact that they were previously read to parents and so have a mysterious life of their own.

There is a plethora of books for children on the market. How does a good grandparent choose? Here are some suggestions.

Keep books for the very young bright and simple with few words and above all with humour. Children love to laugh.

Books for the bath are made of plastic, with very simple pictures of familiar objects and animals; board books have pages that are easy to turn (and difficult to tear), again with very simple pictures; pop-up books are great fun – just a little frightening at first, so give the children time to touch the paper and understand that it is just pretend; and of course there are always nursery rhyme books – both you and your grandchild can chant or sing the rhymes and look at the pictures as well.

For toddlers, look for books that let you do things, with a little more 'story' to the pictures. Jokey rhyming books are usually great favourites with this age group, and books of traditional nursery stories are also enjoyed by pre-school children.

Where to find books

Children love choosing their own books, and local bookshops often have a surprisingly good children's section. Book clubs often offer excellent discounts and you can browse at leisure through their catalogues, some of which give helpful reviews or precis the contents of each book.

TWO RHYMES TO TELL YOUR GRANDCHILDREN
(Before they tell them to you)

Grandpapa fell down the drain,
Couldn't scramble out again.
Now he's floating down the sewer,
That's one Grandpapa the fewer.

Grandmama fell off the boat,
Couldn't swim and *wouldn't* float.
Matilda just stood by and smiled,
I almost could have slapped the child.

(Only for grandparents with a sense of humour.)

'Don't teach your granddame to grope her ducks.'
English proverb

GRANDMAMA
MAKES A QUILT

Queen Victoria worked a quilt for her expected
grandson (the son of the Princess Royal and the
future Kaiser) who was born on 27 January 1859:

'Windsor Castle, January 5, 1859
. . . and last my work for the "little individual";
which I have been employed in since September –
and which (with the exception of the marking and
joining the long strips) I have done every stitch of
myself. You know that Mama has very little time and
that I can only work after dinner when we have no
visitors, therefore it was longer about than it
otherwise would have been, but it gave me such
pleasure that I am quite grieved to have finished it.
Many doubted I should get it ready in time. I only
claim its being used in preference to other people's
work as the grandmama has a first claim.'

Letter from Queen Victoria to the Princess Royal

GRANDMA MOSES

One of the most famous grandmothers made a name for herself as a painter when she was already an old lady. Grandma Moses (Anna Mary Robertson Moses) was born on 7 September 1860 in Greenwich, New York. She always loved drawing as a child and would colour her pictures with the juices of berries and grapes.

Anna Mary left her parents' farm at the age of twelve to be a hired girl until she married Thomas Moses in 1887. They farmed in Shenandoah Valley and in 1905 moved to Eagle Ridge, New York. After Thomas died in 1927, Anna went on farming with the help of her youngest son and started creating worsted embroidery pictures. She only started painting when arthritis overtook her.

Grandma Moses' paintings were primitive and brightly coloured: she painted her memories of what she called 'Old Timey' farm life in New York and Virginia, with titles such as 'Over the River to Grandma's House', and she had fifteen one-woman shows in the US and Europe.

Grandma Moses lived until she was 101 and her birthday was commemorated as Grandma Moses Day by the Governor of New York. She died on 13 December 1961.

MY GREAT GRANDPA

When my Grandpa comes home
From the mill,
With ice-cold fingers
And bony, wrinkled face
Sometimes he reads to me
of monsters at sea.
But there is something mysterious about him,
He looks at the tall grandfather clock
Watching the pendulum
Swing to and fro
And the long hands of the clock reach to
stab the numbers like daggers.

Paul Leipnik (aged 10),
from Young Words 1985 (Macmillan)

THINGS TO DO WITH YOUR GRANDCHILDREN

Grandparents can offer something really worthwhile by sharing their own skills and interests with their grandchildren. One grandparent makes and paints paper butterflies, fixes them to specially selected grass stalks and sells them to local shops. She has commissioned her grandchildren to find the grasses and select the stalks, taken them to several butterfly farms and encouraged them to help her breed

enormous tropical moths from pupae, encouraging them to gather the food which the caterpillars need in order to survive.

Grandparents may be the best people to teach traditional crafts – knitting and crochet and weaving are obvious ones. The Bishop of Leicester, Richard Rutt, was taught to knit by his grandfather who was the village blacksmith. Richard Rutt has collected old books on the history of knitting and numerous knitting patterns and has even written a book, *The History of Hand Knitting* (Batsford), all due to his knitting grandfather.

One grandchild remembers being taught how to tie knots by her sailor grandfather. Another was taught how to set up a fishing rod and line with the correct weights and floats for various fishes; how to cast the line; how to find caddis worms for bait, pulling them out of their carefully constructed camouflage, and seed the riverbed in likely spots for the next day's angling; how to make artificial flies; and how not to be squeamish when pulling a large grub – taken from a coffee tin squirming with a jumble of fat white maggots among smelly meal – on to a hook, and how to hook a worm so that it couldn't escape but still wiggled tantalisingly.

Sometimes grandparents are the ones with the time and patience to teach children a vital skill such as swimming. One grandparent took her grandchildren to the baths every day for two weeks during the summer holidays, something most parents would probably not have the time to do.

The wise grandparent will keep in a drawer modelling material, paper, felt pens, scissors, bits of felt and other fabrics, adhesive, puzzles, packs of cards, scrap books, dice, counters and other interesting objects which the children are allowed to play with but which they might not find at home such as marbles, a solitaire board and old-fashioned board games. If you are a country grandparent, keep a selection of little field books for fine days (on insects, butterflies, birds, wild flowers, grasses, pond life, trees) to take on walks in field or garden, hedgerow or ditch. You don't have to be a 'striding' grandparent – a gentle amble is probably better for looking at things.

Always remember to take a magnifying glass.

If you take your grandchildren to museums or exhibitions, choose ones you will enjoy yourself so that they will catch a little of your enthusiasm. Encourage them to paint or draw what they see.

Rhyme and movement games are fun and repetition of the rhymes is part of that fun. Children learn a great deal through performing rhymes – even the most simple finger-play demands that children think about co-ordination. And much more can be learned with action-play such as jumping, hopping and skipping.

Walking game

Can you walk on tiptoe
As softly as a cat?
And can you stamp along the road,
Stamp stamp stamp, like that?
Can you gallop round about like a horsey prancer?
Or glide about so gracefully like a ballet dancer?

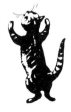

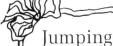

Jumping

Feet together, standing still
I can jump, I will! I will!
Feet together, here I go
Jumping fast, jumping slow.

John Middlecombe

Old John Middlecombe lost his cap (*hands to head*)
He couldn't find it anywhere, the poor old chap
(*search for hat*)
He walked down the high street (*stroll round room*)
And everybody said
'Silly old John Middlecombe –
You've got it on your head' (*hands on head again*).

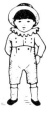

The wheels on the bus

The wheels on the bus go round and round (*hands round and round each other*)
Round and round, round and round
The wheels on the bus go round and round
All day long.

The bells on the bus go ding a ling a ling,
Ding a ling a ling, ding a ling a ling
The bells on the bus go ding a ling a ling
All day long.

The dog on the bus goes yap yap yap . . . etc.
(*Sing to the tune of 'Merrily We Roll Along'.*
Improvise as much as you like: children love to think up their own actions and sounds.)

Tallest tree

Up into the tallest tree (*hold up one arm for tree*)
Who should climb but little me (*two fingers of other hand creep up arm*).
Right to the top, but I couldn't get down (*keep fingers on top of arm*)
So I called to my Grandma
'GRANDMA, GRANDMA'
But Grandma was in town
So I curled myself into a ball (*make a fist*)
and rolled myself down.

Counting game

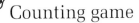

Five little fingers walked over my lap,
One became tired and stopped for a nap.

Four little fingers walked across my knee,
One fell off and that left three.

Three little fingers dancing all around,
One got lost – only two were found.

Two little fingers go up my arm for fun,
One couldn't make it – now there's only one.

One little finger, left all alone,
Cried and cried until the others came home.

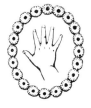

My lady

Here's my lady's knives and forks (*interlace fingers, palms up*)
Here's my lady's table (*turn hand with interlaced fingers down*)
Here's my lady's looking glass (*put up two little fingers, tips together*)
And here's the baby's cradle (*put up forefingers together as little fingers and rock the cradle*).

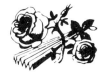

'The grandsire buys, the father builds, the son sells and the grandson begs.'

Scottish proverb

DOMBEY AND
GRANDCHILDREN

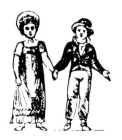

Autumn days are shining and on the sea-beach there are often a young lady, and a white-haired gentleman. With them, or near them, are two children: boy and girl. And an old dog is generally in their company.

The white-haired gentleman walks with the little boy, talks with him, helps him in his play, attends upon him, watches him, as if he were the object of his life. If he be thoughtful, the white-haired gentleman is thoughtful too; and sometimes when the child is sitting by his side, and looks up in his face, asking him questions, he takes the tiny hand in his, and holding it, forgets to answer. Then the child says:

'What, grandpapa! Am I so like my poor little uncle again?'

'Yes, Paul. But he was weak, and you are very strong.'

'Oh yes, I am very strong.'

'And he lay on a little bed beside the sea, and you can run about.'

And so they range away again, busily, for the white-haired gentleman likes best to see the child free and stirring; and as they go about together, the story of the bond between them goes about, and follows them. But no one, except Florence, knows the measure of the white-haired gentleman's affection for the girl. That story never goes about. The child herself almost wonders at a certain secrecy he keeps in it. He hoards her in his heart. He cannot bear to see a cloud upon her face. He cannot bear to see her sit apart. He fancies that she feels a slight, when there is none. He steals away to look at her, in her sleep. It pleases him to have her come and wake him in the morning. He is fondest of her and most loving to her, when there is no creature by. The child says then, sometimes;

'Dear grandpapa, why do you cry when you kiss me?'

He only answers, 'Little Florence! Little Florence!' and smoothes away the curls that shade her earnest eyes.

Charles Dickens, from *Dombey and Son*

GRANDCHILDREN TO STAY

Having your grandchildren to stay is a great treat but is even more enjoyable if you prepare the house for them first. It is easy, once one's own children have grown up, to forget just what it's like having children about the place.

For safety's sake

* Move all valuables and breakables out of reach.
* Put *all* medicines in a locked bathroom cabinet – that includes anything you might normally keep in your handbag, and even innocuous-seeming things such as vitamin pills.
* Household chemicals and cleaners are poisonous. Put them away in a cupboard and seal the doors with sticky tape.
* Cover electric sockets with sticky tape.
* Keep all flexes and electric leads out of reach and keep pan handles turned inwards when you are cooking. Children are often much quicker in their reactions than their grandparents and can reach dangerous items in the twinkling of an eye.

* Don't cover tables with dangling tablecloths that can be pulled off, possibly bringing scalding-hot drinks or food with them.
* Don't allow your grandchildren to play with your cat or dog, who may not be used to children.

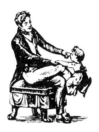

Emergency things to do

Grandparents often find themselves at a loss for toys when grandchildren come to stay. If you find time hanging heavily, here are some things the grandchildren may enjoy doing but which don't require much equipment.

PLAY DOUGH: Mix together a cup of flour, a cup of salt, 2 tablespoons of vegetable oil, some food colouring if you like, and a third to half a cup of water (enough to give a workable dough). A teaspoon of alum or glycerine added to the mixture will keep it damp for longer. Store the dough in a plastic bag in the fridge.

The shaped dough can be baked in a cool oven for several hours, then painted with poster or acrylic paints and glazed with nail varnish.

POTATO PRINTING: Inexpensive, satisfying and fun! Cut a potato in half and carve out a pattern – an animal, a Christmas tree, a face, or just an abstract shape. Dip it in ink or brush with paint, and press down on to fabric or paper.

SPROUTING SEEDS: If your grandchild is staying for a week or more, you can grow some sprouting seeds to be taken back home. Mustard and cress can be grown inside an eggshell – paint a face on the shell, and as it grows the cress will become its hair! Fill the shell with earth or a bit of cloth, sow the seeds and keep them well watered.

HAND SHADOWS: Granddads are often very good at these. You will need to get your hand between a good, bright light and the wall. By putting your fingers and thumb together you can make a quacking duck, a wolf, a rabbit, a dog, and so on. Children like it when you make up a story to go with the shadows.

Tears at bedtime

Your grandchild may show signs of homesickness, particularly in the evenings. Here some kind of bedtime ritual will be welcomed.

* A warm bath is relaxing and fun, especially if you have something the child can use as a boat.
* A hot milky drink is often very comforting.
* A chat about the child's mum and dad will usually help. One of the worst fears a child has is of not understanding what is going on.
* Writing a letter to the absent parents may be a soothing occupation. Preferably include a picture of a local landmark or somewhere visited during the child's stay.
* A bedtime story is always acceptable.
* A tape of nursery rhymes for singing along to is a cheering alternative to a lullaby for a slightly older child.
* Children may be comforted if you give them a special present during the day which they can take to bed with them. This might be anything from a toy car to a piece of your own jewellery, depending on the child's tastes.

SOME TRADITIONAL TREATS

Melting Mouthfuls

3 oz (75 g) soft margarine
2 eggs, beaten
4 oz (100 g) self-raising flour
1 level teaspoon baking powder
3 oz (75 g) caster sugar
1 tablespoon milk
4 oz (100 g) icing sugar
lemon juice
'hundreds and thousands' to decorate

Put the margarine, eggs, flour, baking powder, sugar and milk in a bowl and beat well until thoroughly mixed. Spoon the mixture into petit fours cases – do not quite fill them. Bake at 350°F/180°C/gas mark 4 for 15–20 minutes, until risen and honey-brown, then cool on a cake rack.

When the cakes are cool, add enough lemon juice to the icing sugar to give a spreading consistency. Spoon a little on top of each cake and spread out with the back of a spoon. When almost set, top with some 'hundred and thousands'.

Makes about 50 tiny cakes

Granddad's Quick Chocolate Crispies

All you need are some cornflakes or rice crispies and some plain chocolate or cooking chocolate. Put the chocolate in a basin over a saucepan of hot water and let it melt. Remove the basin from the heat and stir in the cornflakes or rice crispies, mixing them in well so that they are completely covered in chocolate. Set out some paper cases on a tray and put a spoonful of the mixture into each one. Leave the crispies to set for about 5 minutes.

Make sure you have a bib and a damp sponge ready: these are *lovely* and messy to eat!

'Don't teach your grandmother to sup sour milk.'

English proverb

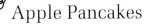

Apple Pancakes

5 oz (150 g) flour
2½ teaspoons baking powder
¼ teaspoon salt
1 egg
½ pint (300 ml) milk
8 oz (225 g) grated cooking apple
melted butter for frying
caster sugar to serve

Sift the flour with the baking powder and salt, and add the egg and milk to make a batter (there is no need to leave it to stand). Add the apple. Lightly grease a griddle or heavy frying pan with some of the butter and cook the pancakes until golden brown on both sides. Serve hot, sprinkled with sugar.

'Don't teach your grandmother to suck eggs.'

English proverb

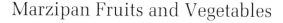

Marzipan Fruits and Vegetables

4 oz (100 g) ground almonds
8 oz (225 g) caster sugar
1 egg white, whisked
vanilla essence
food colourings

Mix together the almonds, caster sugar, egg white and
a few drops of vanilla essence until you have a stiff
paste. Take small quantities and shape them into
oranges, apples, carrots and so on, then paint them
with suitable food colourings. (You can make
marzipan potatoes and nuts by rolling the shapes in
cocoa to colour them brown.)

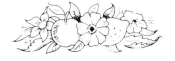

Real Flower Cake and Pudding Decorations

6 oz (175 g) sugar
4 fl oz (120 ml) water
food colouring
fresh flowers (violets, primulas or sweet peas work
very well)
sifted icing sugar for sprinkling

Heat the sugar and water slowly in a saucepan until
the mixture boils; keep boiling until a little of the
mixture forms a soft ball when dropped into cold
water. Remove from the heat and allow to stand until
lukewarm.

Add a few drops of food colouring to the mixture
to match your chosen flowers. Paint the mixture on
each petal, making sure to cover all the surfaces;
when dry, paint on another coat. Sprinkle the flowers
lightly with icing sugar and leave them to dry. Store
in a cool, dry place.

Lemon and Acid Drops

1½ lbs (675 g) loaf sugar
½ pint (300 ml) water
½ teaspoon cream of tartar
lemon essence
1 dessertspoon tartaric acid
sifted icing sugar

Boil the sugar, water and cream of tartar until the
mixture turns a pale yellow colour. Add the lemon
essence to taste and turn on to an oiled slab. Sprinkle
on the tartaric acid and work it in well.

As soon as the mixture is cool enough to handle,
form into thin rolls. Cut off short pieces with a pair of
kitchen scissors and mould into 'drop' shapes with
your hands (children love this bit). Coat with icing
sugar and leave to dry completely, then store in an
airtight tin or plastic box.

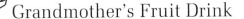

Grandmother's Fruit Drink

2 oranges
2 pints (1.2 litres) boiling water
2–3 lbs (900 g–1.3 kg) sugar
1 oz (25 g) tartaric acid

Finely chop the oranges, put them in a large jug or bowl and pour over the boiling water. Mix in the sugar. Leave for 24 hours, then add the tartaric acid dissolved in a little warm water. Stir well and serve diluted to taste.

This fruit drink will keep for a week or two in a cool place. If you like, replace one or both of the oranges with grapefruit.

'To know a girl really well, examine her grandmother.'

Thai proverb

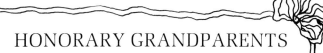

HONORARY GRANDPARENTS

In most societies grandparents have been respected for their experience and wisdom. But in the industrial West where families are often split up, grandchildren and grandparents may hardly ever see each other. This leaves a whole dimension out of both their lives and has inspired the creating of 'honorary' grandparents and other ways of integrating the elderly into the infrastructure of society.

The 'Grandperson Project' was started in the 1970s in Ann Arbor, Michigan, where a sensitive child stabbed and almost killed a classmate in Carol Tice's art class. Ms. Tice wondered why a child would stab another child. In her search for an answer she spent two months riding on school buses with the children and came to the conclusion that the problem lay in the fact that the children did not care for one another.

She felt that what each child needed in the school community was to have someone care for him or her and someone for him or her to care about. The people who would have time for this were older adults – in other words, grandparents, whom she called 'grandpersons'. So she started the 'Grandperson Project'. The scheme relies on grants from health and welfare bodies, from educational bodies, and small contributions from the Association of Elementary School Administrators and other organisations. It was soon followed up in Canada with the Intergenerational Teaching-Learning Communities of Frontenac County, Ontario.

Each grandperson has a skill or craft to share with a group of three, four or five children. On introductory day, grandpersons show and speak of their crafts and students indicate their first, second, and third choices, on the basis of which the classroom teacher assigns them to a group. Though crafts and skills are taught and learned, the most significant development has been the mutual love of child for grandperson and vice versa. Handicrafts have included knitting, embroidery, woodworking, rug hooking, crocheting, sign writing, basket weaving, whittling, coat-hanger covering, artificial flower making, fresh flower arranging, quilting, sewing of rag dolls and pot holders, and making of tiny shell necklaces or bracelets, shell pictures, marionettes and puppets.

The participating grandpersons, who range in age from 55 to 90, are the happiest group of senior citizens conceivable. They make friends, have fun, and enjoy the young. One of them described the project as being a delightful experience. 'To see those bright little faces on the children each Wednesday as I enter the classroom and their enthusiasm literally exploding is very rewarding. I am not sure how much I taught the children in the art of crocheting or crafts, but in five short weeks it is hard to believe the closely established relationship.'

One young student wrote of a 90-year-old grandperson 'He's my friend' and another asked a senior citizen, during her second visit: 'Can I call you Grandma?'

'Judging by the buzz of discussion during the six sessions, I'm sure the seniors are pleased at the many young friends and admirers they have made as well,' said a teacher. 'For the past five weeks, Wednesday afternoons have been the highlight of the school week. The children count off the days until *their* grandperson returns.'

'The property of the grandfathers will come to an end, but the craft of the hands will remain.'

Moorish proverb

THE INCREDIBLE
BOUNCING MAN

Bouncing in and out of
Death's reach, as if he were on elastic.
My Grandad.
'Stand by your beds! Here comes Grandad!'
A permanent smile engraved on his face,
Walking stick in one hand, pint glass in the other.

But annually, at Christmas time, he goes that little bit
Too far, enjoys himself just too much,
Drains his seemingly eternal energy source,
And always ends in hospital.
The family sit round his bed,
Drips sustain his energy and blood level.
His eyes are closed.
The nurses have given up.
Tears form.
Grandad is deathly white, mouth open, just
breathing.
But by the end of that week he is always better.
Four heart attacks, three years of nearly dying at
Christmas,
Two weeks to live in 1960 and twenty years of chain
smoking:
He would never give in to septicaemia.

He's always back, drinking, eating and most of all
talking.
With eighty-two years behind him and countless
years in front,
Causing scandals in his old people's home,
Asking if widows can come and stay with him.
My Grandad is unique.
And wonderful.

Andrew Darley (aged 13),
from *Young Words 1986* (Macmillan)

'Grandmother' was the slang term for the big
Howitzers operated in France by the Royal Marine
Artillery in the First World War.

MORITURI SALUTAMUS

It is too late! Ah nothing is too late
Till the tired heart shall cease to palpitate.
Cato learned Greek at eighty; Sophocles
Wrote his grand Oedipus and Simonides
Bore off the prize of verse from his compeers
When each had numbered more than four-score
years . . .
Chaucer, at Woodstock with the nightingales,
At sixty wrote the Canterbury Tales:
Goethe at Weimar, toiling to the last,
Completed Faust when eighty years were past.
These are indeed exceptions; but they show
How far the gulf-stream of our youth may flow
Into the artic regions of our lives . . .
For age is opportunity no less
Than youth itself, though in another dress
And as the evening twilight fades away
The sky is filled with stars, invisible by day . . .

                    Henry Wordsworth Longfellow